"Forever Fit:Thriving at 40+-Navigating Work and an Active Lifestyle with Wisdom and Vitality"

Introduction:

Acknowledging the unique challenges faced by individuals over 40 in balancing work and an active lifestyle

Balancing work and an active lifestyle is a juggling act that can be especially challenging for individuals over 40. This chapter will address and acknowledge the unique challenges faced by individuals in this age group as they strive to maintain both a successful career and a healthy, active lifestyle.

1. Increased Responsibilities:
- Individuals over 40 often have more significant responsibilities in their careers, as they may hold senior positions or have additional commitments.
- Balancing these increased work responsibilities with maintaining an active lifestyle requires careful time management and prioritization.
- Tips for delegating tasks, setting boundaries, and finding a healthy work-life integration.

2. Declining Energy Levels:
- With age, energy levels tend to decline, making it more challenging to engage in physical activities after long days at work.
- Strategies for managing fatigue and finding ways to incorporate exercise into daily routines, such as early morning workouts or active lunch breaks.

3. Potential Health Issues:
- As individuals age, they may face health challenges that can impact their ability to maintain an active lifestyle.

- Acknowledging and addressing these health issues, whether chronic or age-related, is crucial in finding suitable physical activities and working with healthcare professionals to create a balanced routine.

4. Changing Recovery Time:
- Recovery time tends to increase with age, making it necessary to allow more time for rest and recuperation.
- Understanding the importance of proper rest and recovery in avoiding burnout and preventing injuries.
- Strategies for incorporating activities that promote relaxation, such as yoga or meditation, into a busy schedule.

5. Financial Obligations:
- Individuals over 40 often have more financial obligations, such as mortgages, education expenses for children, or retirement planning.
- Balancing work and an active lifestyle may require finding affordable fitness options or exploring activities that can be done without significant financial burden.

6. Emotional Well-being:
- Balancing work and an active lifestyle can take a toll on emotional well-being, especially as individuals face midlife transitions and personal growth.
- Prioritizing self-care, seeking support from loved ones, and considering therapy or counseling to navigate emotional challenges.

Acknowledging the unique challenges faced by individuals over 40 in balancing work and an active lifestyle is vital for designing strategies that promote overall well-being. By recognizing the increased responsibilities, declining energy levels, potential health issues, changing recovery time, financial obligations, and emotional well-being, individuals can make informed decisions and prioritize their health and happiness. Finding a balance that works for them will contribute to a fulfilling and rewarding life in both their personal and professional spheres.

Emphasizing the importance of maintaining physical and mental well-being in this stage of life

In addition to acknowledging the challenges faced by individuals over 40 in balancing work and an active lifestyle, it is crucial to emphasize the importance of maintaining physical and mental well-being during this stage of life. Here are some key points to consider:

1. Physical Health:
- Regular exercise and physical activity are essential for maintaining overall health and preventing age-related conditions.
- Engaging in activities that promote cardiovascular health, strength, flexibility, and balance can help individuals stay fit and active.
- Prioritizing regular check-ups with healthcare professionals to address any potential health issues and receive guidance on suitable physical activities.

2. Mental Well-being:
- Balancing work and an active lifestyle can be mentally taxing, especially as individuals navigate the challenges of midlife.
- Engaging in activities that promote mental well-being, such as mindfulness, meditation, or hobbies that bring joy and relaxation, is crucial.
- Seeking support from friends, family, or professionals to navigate any emotional or psychological challenges that may arise.

3. Self-Care:
- Individuals over 40 must prioritize self-care to maintain physical and mental well-being.
- This includes ensuring adequate sleep, practicing stress management techniques, and nourishing the body with a balanced diet.
- Taking time for oneself, whether it's engaging in hobbies, pursuing personal interests, or simply enjoying downtime, is essential for rejuvenation.

4. Work-Life Integration:
- Rather than viewing work and an active lifestyle as separate entities, striving for a healthy work-life integration is key.
- Setting boundaries and creating a schedule that allows for both work commitments and time for physical activity and personal pursuits.

- Recognizing that a well-rounded life includes both professional success and personal fulfillment.

5. Long-Term Benefits:
- Investing in physical and mental well-being over 40 can have long-term benefits for overall health and quality of life.
- Maintaining an active lifestyle can help reduce the risk of chronic diseases, improve cognitive function, boost mood, and increase longevity.
- Prioritizing self-care and well-being can lead to increased productivity, better work performance, and a greater sense of fulfillment in all aspects of life.

Maintaining physical and mental well-being is of utmost importance for individuals over 40 as they navigate the challenges of balancing work and an active lifestyle. By prioritizing regular physical activity, engaging in activities that promote mental well-being, practicing self-care, integrating work and personal life, and recognizing the long-term benefits, individuals can ensure a fulfilling and healthy life in this stage of life and beyond.

Chapter 1: Reevaluating Priorities and Goals

Reflecting on personal and professional aspirations in light of changing priorities

As individuals enter their 40s and beyond, it is common for priorities to shift and evolve. This stage of life often brings new perspectives, experiences, and responsibilities that can prompt reflection on personal and professional aspirations. Here are some key points to consider:

1. Reevaluating Priorities:
- Individuals over 40 may find themselves reassessing their goals and aspirations in light of changing priorities.
- This may involve reflecting on personal fulfillment, relationships, health, and overall well-being.

- It is essential to take time for self-reflection and consider what truly matters and brings happiness and satisfaction.

2. Personal Aspirations:
- With changing priorities, personal aspirations may shift towards finding a better work-life balance, pursuing hobbies, or focusing on personal growth and self-care.
- This could involve exploring new interests, setting personal challenges, or seeking out experiences that align with individual passions and values.
- Personal aspirations may involve spending more time with loved ones, traveling, or engaging in activities that bring joy and fulfillment.

3. Professional Aspirations:
- The changing priorities of individuals over 40 may also lead to a reevaluation of professional aspirations.
- This could involve seeking greater meaning and purpose in work, pursuing new career paths, or considering a shift towards more flexible or fulfilling work arrangements.
- Professional aspirations may include finding opportunities for growth, mentorship, or leadership roles that align with personal values and aspirations.

4. Balancing Personal and Professional Goals:
- It is crucial to find a balance between personal and professional aspirations to ensure overall well-being and satisfaction.
- This may involve setting realistic expectations, prioritizing self-care, and making conscious choices that align with personal values and long-term goals.
- Open and honest communication with loved ones and employers can help in finding a harmonious balance between personal and professional aspirations.

5. Embracing Change and Adaptability:
- As priorities and aspirations change, it is essential to embrace the process of adaptation and be open to new opportunities and experiences.
- This may involve taking calculated risks, stepping out of comfort zones, and being willing to learn and grow.
- Embracing change can lead to personal and professional growth, increased resilience, and a more fulfilling life overall.

Reflecting on personal and professional aspirations is a natural part of life for individuals over 40. By reevaluating priorities, considering personal and professional aspirations, finding a balance between the two, and embracing change and adaptability, individuals can navigate this stage of life with purpose and fulfillment. It is important to remember that aspirations may evolve over time, and it is never too late to pursue new goals and dreams that align with one's changing priorities.

Identifying areas of life that require more attention and balance

For people over 40, finding balance and paying attention to various areas of life becomes increasingly important. Here are some key areas that may require more attention and balance during this stage:

1. Health and Wellness:
- Physical health: As the body ages, it becomes essential to prioritize regular exercise, proper nutrition, and preventive healthcare to maintain overall well-being.
- Mental health: Managing stress, practicing self-care, and seeking support when needed are crucial for mental well-being.
- Sleep: Adequate sleep is essential for physical and mental health, so ensuring a consistent sleep routine is important.

2. Relationships and Social Connections:
- Family and loved ones: Nurturing relationships with family members, partners, and close friends becomes increasingly important for emotional support and fulfillment.
- Social connections: Maintaining and cultivating friendships, engaging in social activities, and building new connections can enhance overall well-being.

3. Career and Professional Growth:
- Assessing career goals: Reflecting on career aspirations, job satisfaction, and opportunities for growth and advancement can help individuals align their professional lives with their changing priorities.
- Work-life balance: Striving for a healthy work-life balance becomes crucial to avoid burnout and maintain overall well-being.

- Skill development: Continuously updating skills and seeking new challenges can enhance professional growth and open doors to new opportunities.

4. Financial Stability and Planning:
- Retirement planning: Understanding and planning for future financial needs becomes increasingly important as retirement approaches.
- Budgeting and saving: Ensuring financial stability by managing expenses, saving for emergencies, and investing wisely is essential in this stage of life.

5. Personal Growth and Fulfillment:
- Pursuing hobbies and interests: Allocating time for personal passions, hobbies, and activities that bring joy and fulfillment is important for personal growth.
- Lifelong learning: Engaging in continuous learning, whether through formal education or personal development, can enhance personal and professional growth.
- Setting personal goals: Identifying personal goals and working towards them can provide a sense of purpose and fulfillment.

Finding a balance among these areas is key, as neglecting any one of them can lead to dissatisfaction and a lack of overall well-being. It's important to remember that balance will look different for each individual, so it's essential to identify and prioritize the areas that resonate most with personal values and aspirations. Regular self-reflection and adjustments to one's lifestyle can help in achieving a well-rounded and balanced life.

Setting realistic goals that align with the values and aspirations of this life stage

Setting realistic goals that align with the values and aspirations of people over 40 involves taking into account their life experiences, current responsibilities, and future aspirations. Here are some tips for setting goals at this life stage:

1. Reflect on personal values: Consider what is most important to you at this stage of life. Reflect on your values, priorities, and what brings you fulfillment. This will help you set goals that align with your core beliefs and aspirations.

2. Consider life experiences and achievements: Take stock of your past accomplishments and experiences. Assess what you have learned and how you can leverage those experiences to set meaningful goals that build on your strengths and expertise.

3. Evaluate current responsibilities: Assess your current commitments and responsibilities, such as family, career, and personal obligations. Consider how these factors may impact your ability to pursue certain goals, and find a balance between your aspirations and your existing commitments.

4. Be specific and measurable: Set clear and specific goals that can be measured. Instead of a vague goal like "improve my health," be more specific by setting a goal like "exercise for 30 minutes, five days a week" or "reduce daily sugar intake to less than 25 grams."

5. Break down goals into smaller steps: Large goals can be daunting, so break them down into smaller, actionable steps. This allows you to track progress, maintain motivation, and celebrate achievements along the way.

6. Set realistic timelines: Consider the time and resources required to achieve your goals. Set realistic timelines that consider your other commitments and obligations. This helps to reduce stress and allows for a more sustainable approach.

7. Be adaptable and flexible: Life is unpredictable, and circumstances may change. Be willing to adjust and modify your goals as needed while staying true to your values and aspirations. This allows for a more realistic and resilient approach to goal setting.

8. Seek support and accountability: Share your goals with trusted friends, family members, or mentors who can provide support and hold you accountable. Consider joining support groups or seeking professional guidance to help you stay motivated and on track.

Remember, setting goals is a personal process, and what works for one person may not work for another. The key is to set goals that are meaningful, realistic, and aligned with your values and aspirations, while also being adaptable to life's changes.

Chapter 2: Nurturing Physical Health

Understanding the physical changes that occur with age and their impact on an active lifestyle

As people age, various physical changes occur that can impact an active lifestyle. It's important to understand these changes and adapt accordingly to maintain a healthy and active lifestyle. Here are some common physical changes and their potential impact:

1. Decreased muscle mass and strength: With age, there is a natural decline in muscle mass and strength, known as sarcopenia. This can lead to a decrease in overall physical performance and make activities that require strength, such as weightlifting or intense workouts, more challenging. To address this, focus on resistance training exercises to maintain and build muscle strength.

2. Reduced flexibility and joint stiffness: As we age, joints may become stiffer, and flexibility may decrease. This can affect mobility and make activities like stretching, yoga, or Pilates important for maintaining flexibility and joint health. Regular stretching exercises can help improve flexibility and reduce the risk of injuries.

3. Slower metabolism: Metabolism tends to slow down with age, making weight management more challenging. It's important to maintain a healthy and balanced diet while adjusting calorie intake to match the reduced metabolic rate. Regular exercise, including both cardiovascular and strength training, can help boost metabolism.

4. Decreased bone density: Bone density naturally decreases with age, increasing the risk of osteoporosis and fractures. Weight-bearing exercises, such as walking, jogging, or dancing, can help maintain bone density. Adequate calcium and vitamin D intake are also crucial for bone health.

5. Changes in cardiovascular health: The cardiovascular system undergoes changes with age, including decreased maximum heart rate and reduced cardiac output. Regular

aerobic exercise, such as brisk walking, cycling, or swimming, can help maintain cardiovascular health and reduce the risk of heart disease.

6. Increased recovery time: As we age, the body may take longer to recover from intense physical activities or injuries. It's important to listen to your body and allow for sufficient rest and recovery time between workouts. Incorporating low-impact activities, like swimming or yoga, can also be beneficial for active recovery.

7. Vision and hearing changes: Age-related changes in vision and hearing can impact physical activities. Regular eye and hearing exams are important to address any issues and ensure safety during exercise. Wearing appropriate eyewear and using hearing aids if needed can help maintain an active lifestyle.

Remember, while these physical changes are a part of the aging process, staying active and engaging in regular exercise can help mitigate their impact. It's important to consult with healthcare professionals, such as doctors or physical therapists, to design an exercise program that suits your individual needs and takes these changes into account.

Discussing strategies for maintaining strength, flexibility, and cardiovascular health

Maintaining strength, flexibility, and cardiovascular health is crucial for people over 40 to lead an active lifestyle. Here are some strategies to consider:

1. Strength Training:
   - Incorporate resistance training exercises at least two to three times per week. Focus on compound movements that target multiple muscle groups, such as squats, deadlifts, push-ups, and pull-ups.
   - Gradually increase the intensity and weight as you progress to challenge your muscles and maintain strength.
   - Consider working with a certified personal trainer who specializes in older adults to create a safe and effective strength training program.

2. Flexibility:

   - Engage in regular stretching exercises to improve and maintain flexibility. Focus on both static stretches (holding a stretch for 15-30 seconds) and dynamic stretches (moving through a range of motion).
   - Incorporate activities like yoga or Pilates, which emphasize flexibility and body awareness.
   - Warm-up before exercising and cool down afterward with stretching exercises to prevent muscle stiffness and injury.

3. Cardiovascular Health:
   - Engage in aerobic exercises that elevate your heart rate and increase endurance. Activities like brisk walking, jogging, cycling, swimming, or dancing are excellent choices.
   - Aim for at least 150 minutes of moderate-intensity aerobic exercise per week or 75 minutes of vigorous-intensity exercise.
   - Incorporate interval training, where you alternate between high-intensity bursts and moderate-intensity recovery periods. This can help improve cardiovascular fitness and burn calories.
   - Consider using wearable fitness trackers or heart rate monitors to track your progress and ensure you're exercising in the appropriate heart rate zones.

4. Cross-Training:
   - Include a variety of exercises and activities in your routine to work different muscle groups and prevent overuse injuries.
   - Incorporate activities like yoga, swimming, or Pilates to improve flexibility and balance.
   - Explore outdoor activities like hiking, cycling, or playing sports that engage different muscle groups and add variety to your routine.

5. Proper Nutrition and Hydration:
   - Maintain a balanced diet that includes lean proteins, whole grains, fruits, vegetables, and healthy fats to provide the necessary nutrients for muscle repair and recovery.
   - Stay hydrated before, during, and after exercise to support optimal performance and overall health.

6. Rest and Recovery:

  - Allow for adequate rest and recovery between workouts to prevent overtraining and reduce the risk of injuries.
  - Prioritize sleep, aiming for 7-9 hours per night, as it plays a vital role in muscle recovery and overall well-being.

Remember, it's important to consult with healthcare professionals, such as doctors or physical therapists, before starting or modifying any exercise program, especially if you have any pre-existing conditions or injuries. They can provide personalized guidance based on your specific needs and goals.

Exploring the importance of nutrition, sleep, and stress management in promoting overall well-being

Nutrition, sleep, and stress management play significant roles in promoting overall well-being for people over 40. Here's a closer look at their importance:

1. Nutrition:
  - As we age, our bodies may require different nutritional needs to support optimal health and function. Consuming a balanced diet that includes a variety of nutrient-dense foods is crucial.
  - Prioritize lean proteins, such as fish, poultry, beans, and legumes, to support muscle maintenance and repair.
  - Include plenty of fruits, vegetables, and whole grains to provide essential vitamins, minerals, and fiber.
  - Healthy fats, like those found in avocados, nuts, and olive oil, are important for brain health and reducing the risk of heart disease.
  - Adequate hydration is also essential for overall health, so ensure you're drinking enough water throughout the day.

2. Sleep:
  - Getting sufficient and quality sleep becomes increasingly important as we age. Sleep is crucial for physical and mental health, as it supports various functions, including memory consolidation, hormone regulation, and immune function.

- Aim for 7-9 hours of uninterrupted sleep each night. Establish a consistent sleep schedule, create a comfortable sleep environment, and practice relaxation techniques like deep breathing or meditation to promote better sleep.
- If sleep disturbances persist, it's advisable to consult with a healthcare professional to identify and address any underlying issues.

3. Stress Management:
- Chronic stress can have detrimental effects on overall well-being. It can contribute to increased risk of heart disease, weakened immune function, and mental health issues.
- Engage in stress-reducing activities such as exercise, yoga, meditation, or deep breathing exercises. These practices can help lower blood pressure, reduce anxiety, and promote a sense of calm.
- Prioritize self-care activities that bring you joy and relaxation, such as hobbies, spending time in nature, or connecting with loved ones.
- Seek support from friends, family, or professional counselors if you're experiencing excessive stress or struggling to manage it effectively.

Overall, maintaining a healthy, balanced lifestyle that includes proper nutrition, sufficient sleep, and effective stress management is crucial for promoting well-being in people over 40. It's essential to make these elements a priority and seek professional guidance when needed to ensure your individual needs are met.

Chapter 3: Maximizing Energy and Productivity

Recognizing the importance of energy management in maintaining work-life balance

Energy management is crucial for maintaining work-life balance, especially for individuals over 40 who may have increased responsibilities and demands. Here's why energy management is important and how it can support a healthy work-life balance:

1. Understanding Energy Levels: As we age, our energy levels may naturally decline, making it essential to manage and optimize the energy we have. Recognizing your energy

patterns throughout the day can help you schedule tasks accordingly. For example, if you have higher energy levels in the morning, prioritize important or challenging work during that time.

2. Prioritizing Self-Care: Energy management involves prioritizing self-care activities that replenish and restore your energy. This includes getting enough sleep, engaging in regular exercise, and practicing stress management techniques. By taking care of your physical and mental well-being, you'll have more energy to devote to work and personal life.

3. Setting Boundaries: Establishing clear boundaries between work and personal life helps prevent burnout and promotes a healthy work-life balance. It's important to define specific working hours, limit work-related activities during personal time, and communicate these boundaries to colleagues and family members.

4. Delegating and Outsourcing: As responsibilities increase with age, it becomes crucial to delegate tasks or outsource certain responsibilities. This allows you to focus on activities that align with your strengths and priorities, freeing up time and energy for other aspects of your life.

5. Flexibility and Time Management: Efficient time management is key to balancing work and personal life. Prioritize tasks, eliminate time-wasting activities, and consider flexible work arrangements if possible. This can help create more time and energy for personal activities and relationships.

6. Regular Breaks and Rest: Taking regular breaks throughout the workday and scheduling downtime is vital for maintaining energy levels. Allow yourself to recharge by engaging in activities you enjoy, spending time with loved ones, or simply doing nothing. Rest and rejuvenation are essential for long-term productivity and well-being.

7. Reflecting on Values and Priorities: As people age, their values and priorities may shift. Regularly reflect on what matters most to you and align your choices and commitments accordingly. This helps ensure that your energy is directed towards activities and relationships that bring fulfillment and happiness.

By effectively managing your energy, setting boundaries, prioritizing self-care, and aligning with your values, you can maintain a healthy work-life balance as you age. It's important to remember that balance may look different for everyone, so finding what works best for you is key.

Strategies for optimizing productivity and focus during work hours

Optimizing productivity and focus during work hours is essential for individuals over 40 who may have increased responsibilities and demands. Here are some strategies to help you stay focused and maximize productivity:

1. Establish a Routine: Create a consistent daily routine that aligns with your natural energy levels and preferences. Identify the times of day when you feel most alert and focused, and schedule your most challenging or important tasks during those periods.

2. Prioritize and Plan: Start each day by identifying your top priorities and creating a to-do list. Focus on the most critical tasks first and break them down into smaller, manageable steps. This helps you stay organized and ensures you allocate your time and energy effectively.

3. Minimize Distractions: Minimize distractions in your work environment to maintain focus. This may involve turning off notifications on your phone, closing unnecessary tabs or applications on your computer, and creating a dedicated workspace free from distractions.

4. Take Regular Breaks: Breaks are crucial for maintaining productivity and focus. Incorporate short breaks throughout your workday to rest your mind, stretch, or engage in relaxation techniques. This allows you to recharge and return to your tasks with renewed focus.

5. Use Time-Blocking Techniques: Implement time-blocking techniques to structure your day and allocate specific time slots for different tasks or activities. This helps you stay organized, prevents multitasking, and ensures you give each task the attention it deserves.

6. Practice Mindfulness or Meditation: Regular mindfulness or meditation practices can enhance focus and concentration. Take a few minutes each day to practice deep breathing exercises or mindfulness techniques to calm your mind and improve mental clarity.

7. Optimize Your Workspace: Create an ergonomic and organized workspace that promotes focus and productivity. Ensure your desk is clutter-free, adjust your chair and monitor height for comfort, and have all necessary tools and resources readily available.

8. Stay Physically Active: Regular physical activity has been shown to improve cognitive function and productivity. Incorporate exercise into your routine, whether it's taking a walk during breaks, practicing yoga, or engaging in any form of physical activity that you enjoy.

9. Manage Energy Levels: Recognize when your energy levels are naturally higher or lower throughout the day. Schedule tasks that require more focus and concentration during periods of higher energy, and save less demanding tasks for times when your energy may naturally dip.

10. Practice Self-Care: Prioritize self-care activities outside of work hours to ensure you're physically and mentally well-rested. Get enough sleep, eat a balanced diet, engage in hobbies or activities you enjoy, and spend quality time with loved ones. Taking care of yourself enhances your overall well-being and supports productivity during work hours.

Remember, productivity strategies may vary from person to person, so it's important to find what works best for you. Experiment with different techniques and make adjustments as needed to optimize your productivity and focus as you age.

Techniques for managing energy levels and avoiding burnout throughout the day

Managing energy levels and avoiding burnout is crucial for individuals over 40 to maintain productivity and well-being. Here are some techniques to help you manage your energy and prevent burnout throughout the day:

1. Get Sufficient Sleep: Prioritize getting enough sleep to ensure you wake up feeling refreshed and energized. Aim for 7-9 hours of quality sleep each night by establishing a consistent sleep schedule and creating a sleep-friendly environment.

2. Practice Healthy Eating Habits: Fuel your body with nutritious foods that provide sustained energy throughout the day. Include a balanced mix of whole grains, lean proteins, fruits, vegetables, and healthy fats in your meals. Avoid excessive sugar and processed foods that can lead to energy crashes.

3. Stay Hydrated: Dehydration can cause fatigue and decreased cognitive function. Keep a water bottle nearby and sip water throughout the day to stay hydrated. Limit intake of caffeine and sugary drinks as they can disrupt your energy levels.

4. Take Regular Breaks: Allow yourself regular breaks throughout the day to recharge. Stand up, stretch, or take a short walk to increase blood flow and reduce muscle tension. Use break times to engage in activities that help you relax and clear your mind.

5. Practice Stress Management: Chronic stress can deplete your energy levels and lead to burnout. Implement stress management techniques such as deep breathing exercises, meditation, or mindfulness practices. Find activities that help you unwind and reduce stress, such as listening to music, practicing yoga, or spending time in nature.

6. Prioritize Tasks: Focus on your most important or challenging tasks when your energy levels are highest. Identify your peak productivity periods and schedule demanding tasks accordingly. Delegate or eliminate non-essential tasks that drain your energy and contribute less to your overall goals.

7. Break Tasks into Manageable Chunks: Large, overwhelming tasks can contribute to burnout. Break them down into smaller, more manageable steps. This allows you to make

progress without feeling overwhelmed and helps maintain motivation and energy throughout the process.

8. Practice Time Management: Efficiently manage your time by prioritizing tasks, setting realistic deadlines, and utilizing time management techniques like the Pomodoro Technique (working in focused bursts with short breaks). This helps you maintain focus and prevents overexertion.

9. Foster Positive Relationships: Cultivate positive relationships with colleagues, friends, and family members. Engaging in meaningful social interactions can boost your energy levels and provide emotional support during challenging times.

10. Listen to Your Body: Pay attention to your body's cues and respect your limitations. Pushing yourself excessively can lead to burnout. If you feel overwhelmed or fatigued, take a step back, reassess your workload, and consider adjusting your schedule or seeking support.

Remember, self-care and managing energy levels are ongoing practices. Regularly assess and adjust your strategies to find what works best for you. By prioritizing your well-being and managing your energy effectively, you can maintain productivity and avoid burnout as you age.

Chapter 4: Finding Time for Exercise and Movement

Overcoming time constraints and incorporating exercise into a busy schedule

Incorporating exercise into a busy schedule can be challenging, especially for individuals over 40 who may have many responsibilities. However, it is crucial to prioritize physical activity for overall health and well-being. Here are some strategies to overcome time constraints and incorporate exercise into a busy schedule:

1. Set Realistic Goals: Start by setting realistic exercise goals that you can manage within your schedule. Aim for at least 150 minutes of moderate-intensity aerobic activity or 75 minutes of vigorous-intensity aerobic activity per week, along with strength training exercises twice a week.

2. Prioritize Exercise: Treat exercise as a non-negotiable appointment with yourself. Schedule it into your calendar and make it a priority. Consider it an essential part of your daily routine, just like any other important task.

3. Identify Time Pockets: Look for small pockets of time throughout your day where you can fit in exercise. For example, you can wake up 30 minutes earlier, exercise during your lunch break, or incorporate physical activity into your evening routine. Be creative and resourceful in finding time.

4. Combine Activities: Multitask by combining exercise with other daily activities. For instance, take the stairs instead of the elevator, walk or bike to work if possible, or do squats or lunges while brushing your teeth. Find ways to incorporate movement into your regular activities.

5. Make it a Family Affair: Involve your family or friends in your exercise routine. Take walks or bike rides together, participate in group fitness classes, or go hiking as a family. This not only allows you to spend quality time together but also motivates and holds you accountable.

6. Break it into Smaller Sessions: If it's difficult to find a continuous block of time for exercise, break it into smaller sessions throughout the day. For example, do three 10-minute brisk walks during the day or split your workout routine into two shorter sessions.

7. Maximize Weekends: Utilize weekends to engage in longer exercise sessions. Plan outdoor activities like hiking, swimming, or cycling. This helps compensate for any missed workouts during the week and allows you to enjoy physical activity with more freedom.

8. Use Technology: Take advantage of fitness apps, fitness trackers, or online workout videos that provide flexibility and convenience. These resources offer a wide range of exercises that can be done at home, requiring minimal equipment and time.

9. Stay Active During Sedentary Tasks: If you have a desk job, incorporate movement throughout the day. Take short walking breaks every hour, stretch regularly, or use a standing desk to avoid sitting for long periods.

10. Be Flexible and Adapt: Recognize that your schedule may change from day to day or week to week. Be flexible and willing to adapt your exercise routine accordingly. If you miss a workout, don't get discouraged. Focus on getting back on track as soon as possible.

Remember, even small increments of exercise can make a significant difference in your health. Prioritizing physical activity and finding creative ways to incorporate exercise into your busy schedule will help you maintain a balanced and healthy lifestyle as you age.

Exploring age-appropriate exercise options that promote strength, mobility, and agility

As people age, it becomes essential to choose age-appropriate exercises that focus on strength, mobility, and agility. Here are some exercise options that can promote these aspects for individuals over 40:

1. Strength Training: Incorporate strength training exercises into your routine to maintain muscle mass and bone density. Focus on compound exercises that work multiple muscle groups simultaneously, such as squats, deadlifts, lunges, push-ups, and rows. Start with lighter weights and gradually increase the intensity as you progress.

2. Resistance Band Workouts: Resistance bands are versatile and can provide an effective strength training workout. They are low-impact and can be used for various exercises targeting different muscle groups. Resistance band exercises help improve strength, stability, and flexibility.

3. Yoga: Yoga promotes flexibility, balance, and strength. It can help improve mobility and reduce the risk of injury. Look for yoga classes or online tutorials specifically designed for older adults or beginners. Hatha yoga, gentle flow, or restorative yoga are good options to start with.

4. Pilates: Pilates focuses on core strength, flexibility, and overall body conditioning. It is a low-impact form of exercise that can enhance stability and posture. Pilates exercises can be modified to suit different fitness levels and age groups.

5. Tai Chi: Tai Chi is a traditional Chinese martial art that combines slow, flowing movements with deep breathing and meditation. It improves balance, coordination, and flexibility while reducing stress. Tai Chi is gentle on joints and can be practiced by people of all fitness levels.

6. Cardiovascular Exercises: Engaging in cardiovascular exercises is crucial for heart health and maintaining stamina. Low-impact exercises like walking, swimming, cycling, or using an elliptical machine are gentle on the joints while providing an excellent cardiovascular workout. Aim for at least 150 minutes of moderate-intensity aerobic activity per week.

7. High-Intensity Interval Training (HIIT): For those looking for a time-efficient workout, HIIT can be a great option. It involves short bursts of intense exercise followed by periods of rest or lower-intensity exercise. HIIT workouts can be adapted to different fitness levels and can improve cardiovascular fitness, strength, and metabolism.

8. Balance and Stability Exercises: Include exercises that focus on balance and stability to prevent falls and maintain agility. Standing on one leg, heel-to-toe walk, standing leg swings, and yoga poses like tree pose or warrior III can help improve balance and stability.

9. Functional Training: Incorporate exercises that mimic everyday movements and activities to improve functional fitness. This could include exercises like squats, lunges, step-ups, or carrying weights while walking. Functional training helps improve strength, coordination, and mobility for activities of daily living.

10. Consult with a Professional: If you're unsure about which exercises are appropriate for your age and fitness level, consider consulting with a fitness professional or physical therapist who can design a personalized exercise program tailored to your specific needs.

Remember to listen to your body, start slowly, and gradually increase the intensity and duration of your workouts. It's also important to warm up before exercising and cool down afterward to prevent injuries.

Strategies for making exercise enjoyable and sustainable in the long run

Making exercise enjoyable and sustainable in the long run is crucial for maintaining a consistent fitness routine. Here are some strategies to help individuals over 40 stay motivated and make exercise a lifelong habit:

1. Find Activities You Enjoy: Choose exercises that you genuinely enjoy doing. Whether it's dancing, hiking, swimming, cycling, team sports, or martial arts, engaging in activities that you find fun and fulfilling will make it easier to stick with them in the long run.

2. Set Realistic Goals: Set realistic and achievable goals that are specific, measurable, attainable, relevant, and time-bound (SMART goals). Breaking down big goals into smaller milestones can make them more manageable and provide a sense of accomplishment along the way.

3. Vary Your Routine: Avoid getting bored by mixing up your exercise routine. Try different activities, classes, or workouts to keep things interesting. Incorporating variety not only prevents monotony but also challenges different muscle groups and prevents overuse injuries.

4. Find an Exercise Buddy or Join a Group: Exercising with a friend, family member, or joining a group or fitness class can provide accountability and social support. It can make

workouts more enjoyable and increase motivation. Additionally, group settings often offer a sense of community and can make exercise a social activity.

5. Use Technology and Apps: Utilize fitness apps, wearables, or fitness trackers to monitor progress, set reminders, and track performance. These tools can provide motivation, offer guidance, and help you stay on track with your fitness goals.

6. Make it a Habit: Schedule exercise sessions into your daily or weekly routine. Treating exercise as a non-negotiable appointment can help establish it as a habit. Consistency is key, so try to find a time that works best for you and commit to it.

7. Reward Yourself: Set up a reward system to acknowledge your efforts and achievements. Treat yourself with something you enjoy after reaching specific milestones or completing a certain number of workouts. Rewards can help reinforce positive behavior and make exercise more enjoyable.

8. Listen to Your Body: Pay attention to your body's needs and limitations. Rest and recover when necessary, and don't push yourself beyond your capabilities. Be mindful of any injuries or discomfort and seek professional guidance if needed.

9. Keep Learning: Stay curious and continue learning about fitness and different exercise modalities. Attend workshops, read books or articles, or watch videos related to exercise and wellness. Expanding your knowledge can keep you motivated and open to trying new things.

10. Celebrate Progress: Acknowledge and celebrate your progress, no matter how small. Whether it's reaching a new fitness milestone, improving flexibility, or noticing increased energy levels, give yourself credit for the positive changes you experience through exercise.

Remember, the key is to find activities that you genuinely enjoy and make exercise a part of your lifestyle. It's not just about short-term goals but about creating sustainable habits that promote health and well-being in the long run.

Chapter 5: Mental and Emotional Resilience

Addressing the unique psychological challenges faced by individuals in their 40s and beyond

As individuals enter their 40s and beyond, they may face unique psychological challenges that can impact their motivation and commitment to exercise. Here are some strategies to address these challenges:

1. Embrace Change: Embrace the idea that change is a natural part of life. Accepting and adapting to the physical and psychological changes that come with age can help individuals maintain a positive mindset and approach to exercise.

2. Focus on Health and Well-being: Shift the focus from purely aesthetic goals to overall health and well-being. Recognize that exercise is not just about appearance but also about maintaining physical and mental health, preventing chronic diseases, and improving quality of life.

3. Practice Self-Compassion: Be kind and compassionate towards yourself. Avoid self-criticism and negative self-talk related to age-related changes. Embrace self-acceptance and celebrate the wisdom and experience that come with getting older.

4. Set Realistic Expectations: Adjust expectations to align with age-related changes in physical abilities. Recognize that it may take longer to achieve certain fitness goals or recover from intense workouts. Setting realistic expectations can prevent frustration and discouragement.

5. Prioritize Recovery and Rest: Recovery becomes increasingly important as individuals age. Incorporate rest days, adequate sleep, and recovery strategies such as stretching, foam rolling, and relaxation techniques into your exercise routine. Listen to your body and give it the time it needs to recover.

6. Seek Professional Guidance: Consult with a healthcare professional or certified fitness expert who specializes in working with older adults. They can provide personalized guidance, address concerns, and design exercise routines that are safe and effective for your age and fitness level.

7. Find Meaning and Purpose: Connect exercise with your personal values and passions. Consider how staying active and fit aligns with your life goals and gives you a sense of purpose. Engaging in exercise activities that have personal significance can enhance motivation and satisfaction.

8. Practice Mindfulness: Incorporate mindfulness into your exercise routine. Pay attention to the sensations in your body, focus on the present moment, and cultivate gratitude for what your body is capable of. Mindfulness can help reduce stress, enhance the enjoyment of exercise, and improve overall well-being.

9. Build a Support Network: Surround yourself with supportive and like-minded individuals. Join fitness groups, seek out exercise buddies, or participate in online communities focused on fitness and wellness. Having a support network can provide encouragement, accountability, and a sense of belonging.

10. Emphasize Mental Health Benefits: Regular exercise has numerous mental health benefits, including reducing stress, anxiety, and depression. Recognize the positive impact of exercise on mental well-being and prioritize it as a way to support emotional resilience and overall psychological health.

By addressing the unique psychological challenges faced by individuals in their 40s and beyond, it becomes easier to maintain a positive mindset, stay motivated, and make exercise a sustainable part of their lives.

Techniques for managing stress, cultivating resilience, and promoting mental well-being

Managing stress, cultivating resilience, and promoting mental well-being are essential for individuals over 40. Here are some techniques to help achieve these goals:

1. Stress Management Techniques:
   - Practice relaxation techniques like deep breathing, meditation, or progressive muscle relaxation to calm the mind and body.
   - Engage in regular physical exercise, which can reduce stress hormones and promote the release of endorphins, enhancing mood and reducing anxiety.
   - Prioritize self-care activities that you enjoy, such as reading, taking baths, listening to music, or pursuing hobbies, to relax and recharge.
   - Maintain a healthy work-life balance by setting boundaries, delegating tasks, and scheduling downtime for relaxation and leisure activities.

2. Cultivating Resilience:
   - Foster a positive mindset by focusing on gratitude, optimism, and finding silver linings in challenging situations.
   - Develop problem-solving skills to navigate obstacles and overcome adversity effectively.
   - Build a strong support network of friends, family, or support groups to provide emotional support during difficult times.
   - Practice self-compassion and kindness towards yourself, acknowledging that setbacks and mistakes are part of life's journey.

3. Promoting Mental Well-being:
   - Prioritize sleep by establishing a consistent sleep routine, creating a calming bedtime environment, and practicing good sleep hygiene.
   - Engage in activities that promote mental stimulation, such as reading, puzzles, learning new skills, or engaging in intellectually stimulating conversations.
   - Nurture social connections by maintaining relationships, participating in social activities, and seeking emotional support when needed.
   - Consider seeking professional help, such as therapy or counseling, to address any underlying mental health concerns and develop coping strategies.

4. Practice Mindfulness and Mind-Body Techniques:
   - Engage in mindfulness meditation to cultivate present-moment awareness, reduce stress, and enhance overall well-being.

- Incorporate mind-body techniques such as yoga, tai chi, or qigong, which combine physical movement, breath control, and mindfulness to promote relaxation and mental clarity.
   - Practice journaling to reflect on thoughts and emotions, gain perspective, and identify patterns or triggers that contribute to stress.

5. Maintain a Healthy Lifestyle:
   - Follow a balanced and nutritious diet that includes whole foods, fruits, vegetables, lean proteins, and healthy fats to support brain health and overall well-being.
   - Limit the consumption of alcohol, caffeine, and processed foods, as they can negatively impact mood and mental health.
   - Avoid excessive use of technology and screens, as they can contribute to stress and disrupt sleep patterns.
   - Stay socially engaged by participating in community activities, volunteering, or joining clubs or organizations aligned with your interests.

By incorporating these techniques into daily life, individuals over 40 can effectively manage stress, cultivate resilience, and promote their overall mental well-being.

Exploring mindfulness practices and stress reduction strategies tailored to this life stage

Mindfulness practices and stress reduction strategies can be particularly beneficial for individuals over 40. Here are some approaches tailored to this life stage:

1. Mindful Aging:
   - Embrace the concept of mindful aging, which involves accepting the natural changes and transitions that come with getting older.
   - Practice self-compassion and let go of societal expectations and comparisons, focusing instead on personal growth and fulfillment.
   - Engage in mindfulness meditation specifically geared towards aging, such as body scans or loving-kindness meditation to cultivate self-acceptance and compassion.

2. Mindful Movement:

- Engage in mindful movement practices such as yoga, tai chi, or qigong, which can improve flexibility, balance, and overall well-being.
- Choose gentle and restorative yoga practices that are suitable for your physical capabilities and focus on breath awareness and relaxation.
- Incorporate mindful walking or hiking in nature to connect with the present moment and reduce stress.

3. Gratitude and Reflection:
- Cultivate a regular gratitude practice by reflecting on and appreciating the positive aspects of your life, including relationships, experiences, and personal achievements.
- Keep a gratitude journal or practice gratitude meditation to foster a positive mindset and enhance overall well-being.
- Engage in reflective practices, such as journaling or contemplative walks, to gain insight, process emotions, and find meaning in life's experiences.

4. Time Management and Prioritization:
- Develop effective time management skills to reduce stress and maintain a sense of balance.
- Prioritize activities that bring joy, meaning, and fulfillment, while learning to say no to commitments that do not align with your priorities.
- Practice setting boundaries to protect your physical and mental well-being, allowing time for rest, relaxation, and self-care.

5. Social Connection and Support:
- Seek out social activities and connections that bring joy and fulfillment, such as joining clubs, volunteering, or participating in group activities aligned with your interests.
- Nurture relationships with friends, family, and community members, as social support is crucial for mental well-being.
- Consider joining support groups or engaging in group therapy to connect with others who are navigating similar life stages and challenges.

6. Embracing Change and Transitions:
- Develop a mindset of embracing change as a natural part of life, recognizing that transitions can bring growth and new opportunities.

- Practice mindfulness to navigate life transitions, such as retirement, empty nesting, or career changes, by staying present and managing any associated stress or uncertainty.
- Seek support from professionals, such as career coaches or therapists, when facing significant life transitions to help navigate the emotional and practical aspects.

Remember that each individual's journey is unique, and it's essential to find practices and strategies that resonate with you personally. Experiment with different techniques and be open to adapting them to suit your needs as you navigate this life stage.

Chapter 6: Building a Supportive Environment

Engaging friends, family, and colleagues in supporting an active lifestyle

Encouraging friends, family, and colleagues to support an active lifestyle for people over 40 can be a great way to enhance motivation and create a supportive environment. Here are some strategies to engage them:

1. Communicate your goals: Share your desire to lead an active lifestyle and the benefits it brings. Explain why it's important to you and how it positively impacts your physical and mental well-being.

2. Lead by example: Be a role model by consistently engaging in physical activity and making it a priority in your life. When others see your commitment and the positive changes it brings, they may be inspired to join you.

3. Plan active outings: Organize social activities that involve physical activity, such as hiking, biking, or group fitness classes. Invite friends, family, and colleagues to join you and make it a fun and enjoyable experience.

4. Create activity challenges: Set up friendly challenges or competitions with friends, family, or colleagues to encourage everyone to participate in physical activities. This can

include steps challenges, workout challenges, or even signing up for a charity run together.

5. Establish accountability partnerships: Find a workout buddy or an accountability partner who shares similar health and fitness goals. This can help keep you both motivated and committed to staying active.

6. Share resources and information: Share articles, blogs, or videos related to health, fitness, and active living with your friends, family, and colleagues. This can provide them with valuable information and inspire them to incorporate physical activity into their lives.

7. Encourage active breaks: Encourage short breaks during work or social gatherings for stretching, walking, or other physical activities. This can help break up sedentary behavior and promote movement throughout the day.

8. Support and celebrate milestones: Acknowledge and celebrate the achievements of your friends, family, and colleagues as they progress in their active lifestyle journey. Offer encouragement, praise, and celebrate milestones together to foster a positive and supportive atmosphere.

9. Organize group fitness activities: Consider arranging group fitness classes or activities specifically tailored to the needs and interests of your friends, family, or colleagues. This can include yoga sessions, dance classes, or even hiring a personal trainer for a group workout.

10. Be inclusive and flexible: Recognize that everyone has different abilities, preferences, and schedules. Be open to different activities and accommodate different fitness levels and interests to ensure everyone feels included and supported.

Remember, the goal is to create a positive and supportive environment that encourages and motivates everyone to lead an active lifestyle. By involving friends, family, and colleagues, you can foster a sense of community and make the journey towards a healthier and more active life more enjoyable.

Strategies for fostering a supportive network that encourages health and well-being

Building a supportive network that encourages health and well-being for people over 40 is crucial for maintaining motivation and achieving long-term success. Here are some strategies to foster such a network:

1. Form or join a wellness group: Create or become part of a group of like-minded individuals who share a common goal of health and well-being. This group can meet regularly to discuss challenges, share tips, and provide support and encouragement.

2. Use technology and social media: Join online communities, forums, or social media groups dedicated to health and wellness for people over 40. These platforms offer a space to connect with others, share experiences, and gain valuable insights and support.

3. Attend fitness classes or join a sports club: Participating in group fitness classes or joining a sports club can provide opportunities to meet individuals who prioritize health and well-being. Engaging in activities together can build camaraderie and create a supportive environment.

4. Seek professional guidance: Consult with healthcare professionals, such as doctors, nutritionists, or personal trainers who specialize in working with individuals over 40. They can provide personalized advice, guidance, and support in achieving health and well-being goals.

5. Organize wellness challenges: Initiate friendly challenges within your network that focus on various aspects of health, such as nutrition, exercise, or stress management. This can create a sense of camaraderie, healthy competition, and accountability.

6. Share resources and information: Regularly exchange articles, books, podcasts, or videos related to health and well-being with your network. Discuss and reflect on the information together, encouraging ongoing learning and growth.

7. Plan active outings: Organize group walks, hikes, or bike rides with members of your network. Engaging in physical activities together strengthens bonds, provides opportunities for mutual support, and makes staying active more enjoyable.

8. Celebrate milestones and achievements: Acknowledge and celebrate the accomplishments of individuals within your network. Recognize their efforts along their health journey, whether it's losing weight, reaching a fitness goal, or adopting healthy habits. This positive reinforcement fosters motivation and a sense of accomplishment.

9. Be a supportive listener: Actively listen to the challenges and triumphs of others within your network. Offer empathy, understanding, and encouragement. Sometimes, having someone to talk to who understands the journey can make all the difference.

10. Create a culture of positivity and non-judgment: Foster an environment where everyone feels comfortable sharing their experiences, setbacks, and successes without fear of judgment. Encourage a positive and uplifting atmosphere that promotes growth, resilience, and self-acceptance.

Remember, building a supportive network takes time and effort. Nurture these relationships, be a source of support for others, and in turn, you will receive the same support and encouragement. Together, you can create a network that embraces health and well-being for people over 40.

Chapter 7: Adapting to Age-Related Changes

Understanding and accepting the physical limitations and changes that come with age

Understanding and accepting the physical limitations and changes that come with age is crucial when creating a supportive work environment for individuals over 40. Here are a few key points to consider:

1. Education and awareness: Promote education and awareness among employees about the natural physical changes that occur with age. This can help foster empathy and understanding among colleagues, reducing age-related stereotypes or biases.

2. Accommodations and adaptations: Provide necessary accommodations and adaptations to support employees' physical limitations. This could include ergonomic workstations, adjustable desks, or assistive devices to minimize strain and discomfort.

3. Health and wellness programs: Offer health and wellness programs tailored to the needs of mature professionals. These programs can include fitness classes, stress management workshops, or nutrition counseling to support their overall well-being and address age-related health concerns.

4. Flexibility in work arrangements: Consider implementing flexible work arrangements, such as part-time schedules or telecommuting options, to accommodate physical limitations or medical appointments. This flexibility can help employees better manage their health while still fulfilling their work responsibilities.

5. Ongoing training and development: Provide opportunities for continuous skill development and training to ensure that employees can adapt to any physical changes and remain productive in their roles. This can include technology training or professional development programs.

6. Open communication and feedback: Encourage open communication between employees and management to address any challenges or concerns related to physical limitations. Regular feedback sessions can help identify potential areas for improvement and find suitable solutions.

Remember, creating a work environment that embraces and supports the physical changes that come with age can contribute to a more inclusive and productive workplace for individuals over 40.

Strategies for modifying exercise routines and activities to accommodate these changes

Modifying exercise routines and activities to accommodate the physical changes that come with age is essential for individuals over 40 to maintain their fitness and overall well-being. Here are some strategies to consider:

1. Warm-up and cool-down: Prioritize warm-up exercises to prepare the body for physical activity and cool-down exercises to gradually bring the heart rate and breathing back to normal. This helps reduce the risk of injury and muscle soreness.

2. Low-impact exercises: Choose low-impact exercises that are gentler on the joints, such as swimming, cycling, or using an elliptical machine. These activities can provide cardiovascular benefits without placing excessive stress on the body.

3. Strength training: Incorporate strength training exercises to maintain muscle mass and bone density. Focus on lighter weights and higher repetitions to reduce the risk of strain or injury. Resistance bands or bodyweight exercises can also be effective alternatives.

4. Flexibility and mobility exercises: Prioritize stretching and mobility exercises to improve flexibility and joint range of motion. This can help alleviate stiffness and reduce the risk of injury. Yoga, Pilates, and tai chi are excellent options for enhancing flexibility and balance.

5. Listen to your body: Pay attention to any discomfort or pain during exercise. Modify or avoid activities that exacerbate existing conditions or cause excessive strain. It's important to work within your individual capabilities and limitations.

6. Incorporate variety: Engage in a variety of exercises to target different muscle groups and prevent overuse injuries. Mixing up your routine also keeps things interesting and helps you stay motivated.

7. Seek professional guidance: Consult with a qualified fitness professional or a healthcare provider who specializes in exercise for older adults. They can provide personalized advice and guidance tailored to your specific needs and limitations.

Remember, it's crucial to listen to your body, respect your limits, and make adjustments as necessary. By modifying exercise routines and activities, individuals over 40 can continue to enjoy the benefits of regular physical activity while accommodating the changes that come with age.

Exploring alternative forms of physical activity that are gentle yet effective

For individuals over 40 looking for alternative forms of physical activity that are gentle yet effective, there are several options to consider. Here are a few ideas:

1. Yoga: Yoga combines gentle stretching, controlled movements, and deep breathing. It improves flexibility, strength, and balance while promoting relaxation and stress reduction. Look for classes that cater specifically to older adults or those with limited mobility.

2. Pilates: Pilates focuses on core strength, stability, and body awareness. It is a low-impact exercise that can help improve posture, flexibility, and muscle tone. Beginners can start with mat-based Pilates or consider using equipment like the Pilates reformer.

3. Tai Chi: Tai Chi is a slow and flowing martial art that emphasizes gentle movements, balance, and coordination. It promotes relaxation, improves flexibility, and enhances mental focus. Tai Chi can be especially beneficial for older adults as it is low impact and can be adapted to different fitness levels.

4. Water-based activities: Swimming, water aerobics, or aqua jogging are excellent options for low-impact exercise. The buoyancy of water reduces stress on the joints while providing resistance for strength training and cardiovascular benefits. These activities can be particularly helpful for individuals with arthritis or joint pain.

5. Walking: Walking is a simple and accessible exercise that can be tailored to individual fitness levels. It improves cardiovascular health, strengthens muscles, and supports bone health. Consider incorporating walking into your daily routine by taking longer walks, exploring nature trails, or joining walking groups for added motivation.

6. Cycling: Cycling is a low-impact exercise that can be enjoyed outdoors or indoors on a stationary bike. It strengthens the lower body, improves cardiovascular fitness, and is gentle on the joints. Start with shorter distances and gradually increase intensity and duration as your fitness improves.

Remember to listen to your body and start at a comfortable level. If you have any underlying health concerns, it's always a good idea to consult with a healthcare professional before starting a new exercise regimen.

Chapter 8: Embracing Midlife Transitions

Navigating career changes, empty nest syndrome, and other midlife transitions

Navigating career changes, empty nest syndrome, and other midlife transitions can be challenging for people over 40. Here are some suggestions to help you through these transitions:

1. Reflect on your values and goals: Take time to reflect on what is important to you and what you want to achieve in this phase of your life. Identify your passions, skills, and areas for personal growth. This self-reflection will help guide you towards a fulfilling career or new interests.

2. Explore your options: Research different career paths or hobbies that align with your interests and values. Consider taking courses or attending workshops to enhance your skills or learn something new. Networking with professionals in your desired field can provide valuable insights and opportunities.

3. Seek support and guidance: Reach out to career coaches, mentors, or support groups that specialize in midlife transitions. They can provide guidance, help you set goals, and offer valuable advice based on their experiences.

4. Embrace change: Be open to new possibilities and be willing to step out of your comfort zone. Change can be intimidating, but it also presents opportunities for growth and personal development. Embracing change with a positive mindset can lead to exciting new experiences.

5. Take care of yourself: Focus on self-care during these transitions. Prioritize your physical and mental well-being by engaging in activities you enjoy, practicing mindfulness or meditation, and maintaining a healthy lifestyle. This will help you stay motivated and resilient during times of change.

6. Connect with others: Reach out to friends, family, or support groups who may be going through similar transitions. Sharing your experiences and feelings can provide emotional support and a sense of community. Additionally, consider volunteering or joining organizations related to your interests to expand your network and meet new people.

Remember, transitions can take time, and it's important to be patient and kind to yourself during the process. Embrace the opportunity for personal growth and trust that you have the ability to navigate these transitions successfully.

Strategies for finding purpose and fulfillment beyond work and family responsibilities

Finding purpose and fulfillment beyond work and family responsibilities is important for personal growth and overall well-being. Here are some strategies to help you in this journey:

1. Explore your passions and interests: Take time to identify activities or hobbies that bring you joy and fulfillment. It could be anything from art, music, sports, writing,

volunteering, or learning something new. Engaging in activities that align with your passions can provide a sense of purpose and personal fulfillment.

2. Set personal goals: Define what success means to you beyond work and family. Set specific goals that align with your values and interests. These goals could be related to personal development, health and wellness, travel, or making a positive impact in your community. Having clear goals will give you something to work towards and provide a sense of purpose.

3. Embrace lifelong learning: Continuously seek opportunities to learn and grow. Take courses, attend workshops, or pursue further education in areas that interest you. This not only expands your knowledge but also keeps your mind engaged and open to new possibilities.

4. Find meaning through volunteering: Engaging in volunteer work can be a fulfilling way to make a positive impact and find purpose beyond your immediate responsibilities. Look for organizations or causes that resonate with you and offer your time and skills to make a difference in the lives of others.

5. Cultivate meaningful relationships: Build and nurture relationships with like-minded individuals who share your interests and values. Surrounding yourself with supportive and inspiring people can bring fulfillment and a sense of belonging.

6. Practice self-care: Prioritize self-care to maintain your physical, mental, and emotional well-being. Make time for activities that relax and recharge you, such as exercise, meditation, hobbies, or spending time in nature. Taking care of yourself allows you to show up more fully in all areas of your life.

7. Reflect and reassess: Regularly reflect on your journey and reassess your goals and priorities. As you grow and evolve, your sense of purpose may change. Give yourself permission to adapt and adjust your path accordingly.

Remember, finding purpose and fulfillment is a personal journey, and it may take time to discover what truly brings you joy and fulfillment. Be patient with yourself, embrace the process, and keep an open mind to new experiences and opportunities that may come your way.

Exploring new hobbies, passions, and avenues for personal growth

Exploring new hobbies, passions, and avenues for personal growth can be a rewarding and fulfilling experience, regardless of age. Here are some ideas to consider:

1. Try something new: Step out of your comfort zone and try activities or hobbies that you've always been curious about. It could be learning to play a musical instrument, painting, cooking, gardening, photography, dancing, or even joining a local theater group. Exploring new interests can open up a whole new world of possibilities and provide a sense of fulfillment.

2. Learn a new skill: Consider acquiring a new skill or expanding your knowledge in a particular area. You could take up a language course, learn to code, start a blog, or develop your writing skills. Engaging in lifelong learning keeps your mind sharp and helps you stay curious and engaged with the world around you.

3. Engage in physical activities: Prioritize your physical well-being by engaging in activities that promote fitness and health. Try yoga, hiking, swimming, cycling, or any other form of exercise that appeals to you. Regular physical activity not only improves your physical health but also enhances your mental well-being.

4. Volunteer for a cause: Explore opportunities to give back to your community by volunteering for a cause that resonates with you. It could be working with a local charity, mentoring others, or getting involved in environmental initiatives. Volunteering can provide a sense of purpose and fulfillment by making a positive impact on the lives of others.

5. Join clubs or groups: Look for clubs, organizations, or interest groups that cater to your specific hobbies or passions. This could include book clubs, hiking groups,

photography clubs, or any other group that aligns with your interests. Connecting with like-minded individuals allows you to share experiences, learn from others, and foster new relationships.

6. Travel and explore: Plan trips to new destinations, whether near or far. Traveling offers the opportunity to experience different cultures, broaden your perspective, and create lasting memories. It can also push you out of your comfort zone and provide a sense of adventure and personal growth.

7. Prioritize self-reflection: Take time for self-reflection and introspection. Ask yourself what truly brings you joy and fulfillment. Reflect on your values, interests, and aspirations. This self-awareness will guide you in discovering new hobbies and passions that align with your authentic self.

Remember, it's never too late to explore new hobbies, passions, and avenues for personal growth. Embrace the journey, be open to new experiences, and allow yourself the freedom to pursue what brings you joy and fulfillment.

Chapter 9: Sustaining Long-Term Balance and Well-being

Developing a sustainable routine that integrates work and an active lifestyle

Developing a sustainable routine that integrates work and an active lifestyle is key to maintaining a healthy and balanced life, especially for people over 40. Here are some tips to help you create such a routine:

1. Prioritize self-care: Start by acknowledging the importance of self-care. Make sure you allocate time for activities that promote physical and mental well-being, such as exercise, meditation, quality sleep, and healthy eating. Taking care of yourself will give you the energy and mindset needed to excel in both work and an active lifestyle.

2. Plan and schedule: Set aside specific time blocks for work, physical activity, and personal time. Create a schedule that allows for a good balance between these areas. Consider using digital tools or apps to help you stay organized and track your progress.

3. Incorporate physical activity into your day: Find creative ways to include physical activity throughout your day. Instead of sitting for long periods, incorporate short walks or stretching breaks. Consider biking or walking to work if feasible. Schedule regular workouts or fitness classes that you enjoy and commit to them as you would any other important appointment.

4. Make movement a natural part of your routine: Look for opportunities to incorporate movement into your daily activities. Take the stairs instead of the elevator, walk or bike for short errands, or have walking meetings whenever possible. Finding ways to be active throughout the day will help you maintain an active lifestyle without feeling overwhelmed.

5. Set realistic goals: Define achievable goals for both work and physical activity. Break them down into smaller, manageable tasks. This will help you stay focused and motivated. Celebrate your accomplishments along the way, as this will keep you motivated to continue your progress.

6. Find a support system: Surround yourself with like-minded individuals who value an active lifestyle. Join fitness groups, participate in sports leagues, or find workout buddies who can keep you accountable and motivated. Having a support system can make it easier to stick to your routine and provide a sense of community.

7. Practice work-life balance: Establish boundaries between work and personal life. Avoid overworking and make time for activities that bring you joy and relaxation. Engaging in hobbies, spending time with loved ones, and pursuing personal interests should be integral parts of your routine.

Remember, it's important to be flexible and adaptable as life's demands change. Be kind to yourself and adjust your routine as needed. By integrating work and an active lifestyle, you'll create a sustainable routine that promotes overall well-being and allows you to thrive in all areas of your life.

Strategies for maintaining motivation and avoiding stagnation

Maintaining motivation and avoiding stagnation can be challenging at any age, but it becomes even more important as we get older. Here are some strategies to help you stay motivated and avoid stagnation:

1. Set meaningful goals: Start by setting clear and meaningful goals that align with your values and aspirations. These goals can be related to work, personal development, health, relationships, or any other area of life. Having goals gives you something to work towards and keeps you motivated.

2. Break goals into smaller milestones: Break down your larger goals into smaller, achievable milestones. This will make them less overwhelming and easier to track your progress. Celebrate each milestone you achieve, as it will help maintain your motivation and keep you moving forward.

3. Embrace lifelong learning: Never stop learning and challenging yourself. Engage in activities that stimulate your mind, such as reading, taking courses, or learning new skills. This keeps your mind sharp and expands your horizons, preventing stagnation.

4. Try new things: Step out of your comfort zone and try new activities or hobbies. Exploring new interests and experiences keeps life exciting and helps you grow as an individual. It can also lead to new opportunities and connections.

5. Surround yourself with positive influences: Surround yourself with positive, supportive, and like-minded individuals. Seek out mentors, join communities or groups with similar interests, and engage in meaningful conversations. Being around people who inspire and motivate you can have a significant impact on your own motivation and growth.

6. Regularly reassess and adjust: Take time to regularly reassess your goals and progress. Reflect on what is working well and what may need adjustment. Sometimes, our priorities

and interests change over time, and it's important to adapt accordingly. This ensures that you stay on the right path and avoid stagnation.

7. Celebrate successes and practice self-care: Acknowledge and celebrate your achievements, no matter how big or small. Rewarding yourself for reaching milestones can provide a sense of accomplishment and motivation to keep going. Additionally, prioritize self-care activities that rejuvenate and recharge you, such as exercise, relaxation, or pursuing hobbies you enjoy.

8. Find purpose and meaning: Connect with your sense of purpose and find meaning in what you do. Understanding why you do certain things can provide a deeper motivation and sense of fulfillment. Reflect on your values, passions, and the impact you want to make in the world.

Remember that motivation may ebb and flow, and that's normal. It's important to be patient with yourself and stay committed to your overall growth and well-being. By implementing these strategies, you can maintain motivation and avoid stagnation, leading to a fulfilling and vibrant life.

Embracing a holistic approach to well-being that encompasses physical, mental, and emotional health

Embracing a holistic approach to well-being is crucial for people over 40 as it encompasses physical, mental, and emotional health. Here are some key aspects to consider:

1. Physical health: Take care of your body through regular exercise, proper nutrition, and sufficient rest. Engage in activities that promote strength, flexibility, and cardiovascular fitness. Consider incorporating a mix of aerobic exercises, strength training, and activities that improve balance and coordination. It's also important to prioritize sleep and manage stress levels to support overall physical well-being.

2. Mental stimulation: Keep your mind active and engaged through activities that challenge your cognitive abilities. This can include reading, solving puzzles, learning new

skills or languages, playing musical instruments, or engaging in creative hobbies. Continued mental stimulation helps improve memory, focus, and overall cognitive function.

3. Emotional well-being: Pay attention to your emotional health by practicing self-care and managing stress effectively. Engage in activities that promote relaxation, such as meditation, deep breathing exercises, or spending time in nature. Cultivate positive relationships and seek support from friends, family, or professional counselors when needed. Prioritize activities that bring you joy and help you manage emotions effectively.

4. Regular health screenings: Stay proactive about your health by scheduling regular check-ups and screenings recommended for your age group. This includes monitoring blood pressure, cholesterol levels, and getting age-appropriate cancer screenings. Staying on top of preventive measures can help detect and address any potential health issues early on.

5. Social connections: Maintain and nurture social connections as they play a vital role in emotional well-being. Cultivate meaningful relationships with friends, family, and the community. Engage in social activities, join clubs or organizations, and participate in group activities that align with your interests. Social connections provide a support system, reduce feelings of isolation, and contribute to overall happiness and well-being.

6. Mindfulness and stress management: Practice mindfulness techniques to stay present and reduce stress. This can include meditation, deep breathing exercises, journaling, or engaging in activities that promote relaxation and self-reflection. Managing stress is crucial as it directly impacts both mental and physical health.

7. Prioritize self-care: Set aside time for self-care activities that bring you joy and help you recharge. This can include pursuing hobbies, taking up a new hobby or interest, practicing gratitude, enjoying nature, or engaging in activities that promote relaxation and self-reflection. Taking care of yourself is essential for overall well-being.

Remember, a holistic approach to well-being is about creating a balanced and integrated lifestyle that supports your physical, mental, and emotional health. By incorporating these practices into your daily life, you can enhance your well-being and enjoy a fulfilling and vibrant life over 40.

Conclusion:

Recap of key takeaways from the book

Here's a recap of key takeaways for people over 40:

1. Embrace a holistic approach: Focus on your physical, mental, and emotional well-being. Recognize that they are interconnected and prioritize activities that support all three areas of your health.

2. Prioritize physical health: Engage in regular exercise, eat a balanced diet, and get enough rest. Incorporate activities that promote strength, flexibility, cardiovascular fitness, and balance.

3. Stimulate your mind: Keep your brain active by challenging it with activities like reading, puzzles, learning new skills, and engaging in creative hobbies. This helps improve memory, focus, and cognitive function.

4. Take care of your emotional well-being: Practice self-care, manage stress effectively, and engage in activities that promote relaxation. Cultivate positive relationships and seek support when needed.

5. Regular health screenings: Stay proactive about your health by scheduling regular check-ups and age-appropriate screenings. This helps detect and address potential health issues early on.

6. Foster social connections: Cultivate meaningful relationships with friends, family, and the community. Engage in social activities and participate in groups aligned with your interests. Social connections provide support and contribute to overall happiness.

7. Practice mindfulness and stress management: Incorporate mindfulness techniques like meditation, deep breathing, and journaling into your daily routine. Manage stress effectively, as it impacts both mental and physical health.

8. Prioritize self-care: Set aside time for activities that bring you joy and help you recharge. Pursue hobbies, practice gratitude, and engage in activities that promote relaxation and self-reflection.

By embracing these takeaways, you can create a well-rounded and fulfilling life that supports your overall well-being as you navigate your 40s and beyond.

Encouragement to embrace this stage of life with wisdom, vitality, and a commitment to well-being

Embracing this stage of life with wisdom, vitality, and a commitment to well-being is a wonderful mindset. Here's some encouragement for people over 40:

1. Embrace your wisdom: You've gained valuable life experience and wisdom over the years. Use this knowledge to make informed decisions, solve problems, and navigate challenges with confidence. Your wisdom is a powerful asset that can guide you towards a fulfilling and meaningful life.

2. Emphasize self-care: Prioritize your well-being and make self-care a non-negotiable part of your routine. Take time to nurture your physical, mental, and emotional health. This not only benefits you but also allows you to show up as your best self for those around you.

3. Embrace change: Recognize that change is a natural part of life. Embrace it with an open mind and a positive attitude. Embracing change can lead to personal growth, new opportunities, and a greater sense of fulfillment.

4. Stay curious and continue learning: Never stop learning and exploring new interests. Embrace curiosity and seek out new experiences, whether it's through reading, taking up

a hobby, or pursuing further education. This keeps your mind engaged and helps you stay mentally sharp.

5. Cultivate gratitude: Practice gratitude for the blessings and experiences in your life. Appreciate the present moment and find joy in the little things. Cultivating gratitude fosters a positive mindset and enhances overall well-being.

6. Embrace a healthy lifestyle: Prioritize your physical health by adopting healthy habits. Engage in regular exercise, eat nutritious foods, get enough sleep, and manage stress effectively. Taking care of your body allows you to maintain vitality and enjoy an active and fulfilling life.

7. Seek meaningful connections: Surround yourself with positive and supportive people who uplift and inspire you. Foster meaningful relationships and invest time in building connections with loved ones and your community. Meaningful connections provide a sense of belonging and contribute to overall happiness.

Remember, age is just a number, and your 40s and beyond can be some of the most fulfilling and vibrant years of your life. Embrace this stage with enthusiasm, prioritize your well-being, and continue to grow and evolve as an individual. You have the wisdom and vitality to make this stage of life truly remarkable.

Final thoughts on the importance of finding balance and living a fulfilling, active life beyond 40.

Finding balance and living a fulfilling, active life beyond 40 is crucial for overall well-being. Here are some final thoughts on why it's important:

1. Physical health: Maintaining a balanced and active lifestyle helps to improve and sustain physical health. Regular exercise, proper nutrition, and sufficient rest enable you to maintain vitality, reduce the risk of chronic diseases, and increase longevity.

2. Mental well-being: Finding balance and engaging in fulfilling activities promotes mental well-being. It helps to reduce stress, anxiety, and depression, while boosting cognitive function and enhancing overall mental clarity and focus.

3. Personal growth: Living a fulfilling life beyond 40 allows for continuous personal growth. It opens up new opportunities for learning, expanding your skills, and exploring different interests. Embracing new challenges and experiences can lead to self-discovery, increased confidence, and a sense of accomplishment.

4. Quality relationships: Finding balance and living a fulfilling life also involves nurturing and prioritizing relationships. Meaningful connections with loved ones and friends provide emotional support, love, and a sense of belonging. These relationships contribute to happiness, fulfillment, and overall life satisfaction.

5. Role model for others: By embracing balance and living a fulfilling, active life beyond 40, you become a role model for others, inspiring them to do the same. Your actions can motivate and encourage those around you to prioritize their well-being, embrace new experiences, and live life to the fullest.

Remember, finding balance and living a fulfilling, active life beyond 40 is about making intentional choices that align with your values and priorities. It's never too late to start or continue on this journey. Embrace this stage of life with openness, curiosity, and a commitment to your well-being, and you'll discover the joys and rewards of living a truly fulfilling and active life.